KETO DIET FOR BEGINNERS 2019

10 Simple Steps to Keto Success
Easy and Healthy Everyday Ketogenic Diet Recipes
You'll Love

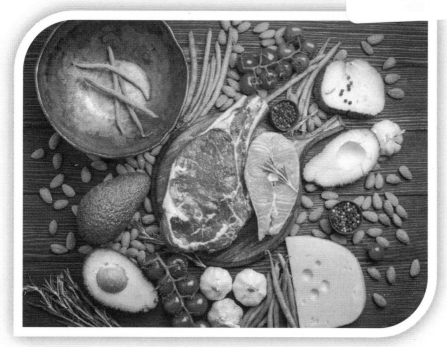

Liam Sandler © 2019

Table of Contents

INTRODUCTION

The ketogenic diet is where you actively go into the state of ketosis by monitoring your diet and lowering your carbs. Ketosis is the state in which your body starts to burn fat because it stops using sugar as its main source of energy. It's a metabolic adaptation which uses stored fat as its source of energy when you're in this state. Of course, it can be difficult to stay in ketosis, which is where your diet is essential. You'll need to keep track of how many net carbs you're consuming.

The standard ketogenic diet allows you to have 5% carbs, 20% protein, and 70% fat. Ideally, you need to keep your net carb intake for a day below twenty carbs, but twenty-three is the cap for an average person. That's exactly what these 30-minute recipes are based on. You'll find they usually have under ten net carbs in each meal, so it's easy to stay full on the ketogenic diet and still reach your weight loss goals.

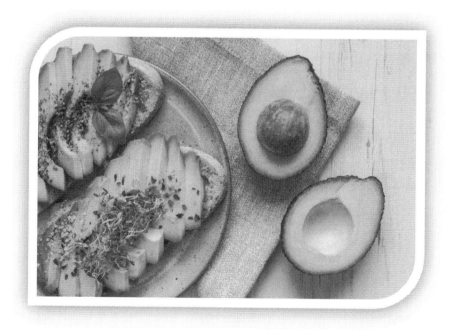

STEPS TO SUCCESS

Now that you know what the ketogenic diet is, and you know you're ready to commit, let's talk about some steps to help you get started.

STEP 1: TAKE AWAY TEMPTATION

If you give into temptation, then you break your diet and therefore ketosis. This will mean that all your work would be for nothing. That's why it's best to remove temptation, which will even help you to commit to exercise! You must view your willpower as a muscle because it'll fatigue as well if you use it too much. If you're constantly battling temptation, it's only a matter of time before you have to give in. for example, if you leave ice cream in the freezer that isn't ketogenic friendly, then you'll be looking at that ice cream each and every time that you open the freezer to get something. It doesn't matter how innocently you're looking at it, eventually you will give in.

So, start by going through your pantry, car snacks, office snacks, refrigerate or any hidden stash of goodies that you have in your house. Make sure to get rid of any non-keto foods. You shouldn't have to test your will power on a daily basis, so leave the heartache in the past. You may need to talk to loved ones, friends or even coworkers to give them a heads up on your dietary changes so they don't accidentally tempt you by offering you something you can't have as well. Keep in mind, that if you live with others, it will be hard to erase all temptation unless they start the ketogenic diet with you, so just avoid it as much as possible.

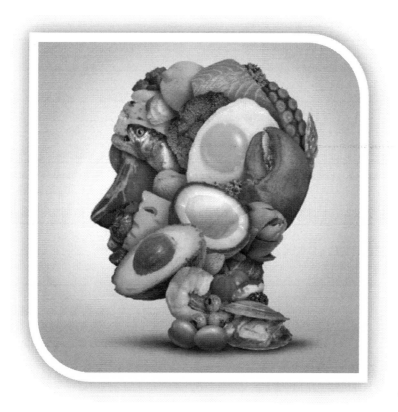

STEP 2: START PLANNING YOUR MEALS

You'll need to plan out your meals at least every few days so that you have the food you need to eat three times a day. This will help to make sure that you aren't ever hungry and tempted by fast food. Meal prepping is also an option, where you plan and cook your meals in advance. Remember that if something is easier, then you're likely to lean towards it. for example, if you know you're going to have a busy week, take a few hours on Sunday to cook a few breakfasts on the go, pack some snack baggies with keto friendly snacks, and maybe even start your week off by making a few lunches or dinners. Either way, you'll at the very least must figure out what you want to eat and what you need to buy to cook your meals properly. Having a plan makes you less likely to make a decision that could break your ketogenic diet.

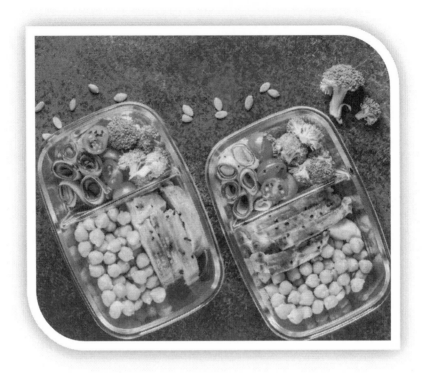

STEP 3: ALWAYS HAVE SNACKS

This isn't just about having snacks in your fridge. You'll need to have snacks on your person as well. After all, most people can just go grab some fries or crackers when they're hungry, but if you're trying to maintain ketosis, you won't be able to. You'll be tempted to cheat during the day. It doesn't matter if you're sitting in the office or you're at your kid's practice. All that matters are that you need keto approved snacks.

Vegetable sticks are a great option, but so are beef jerky, avocados, string cheeses, nuts, seaweed snacks are more. Just have something on hand or at least in your car. You'll want to have snacks that are great on the go. For example, nuts and seeds are a great quick keto friendly snack, but if they're all you use then you'll be getting too much protein. Instead, you should try to carry around some vegetable sticks or seaweed snacks that are great on the go.

STEP 4: MONITOR YOUR PROTEIN

While you're working on sticking to the ketogenic diet, you'll have to monitor your protein intake. You need to keep it a moderate twenty percent of your calories, so that you preserve lean body mass. Otherwise, too much protein will pull you out of ketosis as well, which will ruin your chances for healthy weight loss. You should keep a journal at the beginning of how much protein you're consuming, and in the beginning, you need to avoid protein filled snacks. With each recipe in this book, you have the amount of protein written down. Just think about how much protein you're consuming regarding how many calories you're actually taken in. if you're mindful and have the list in front of you, then you're less likely to actually deviate from the plan.

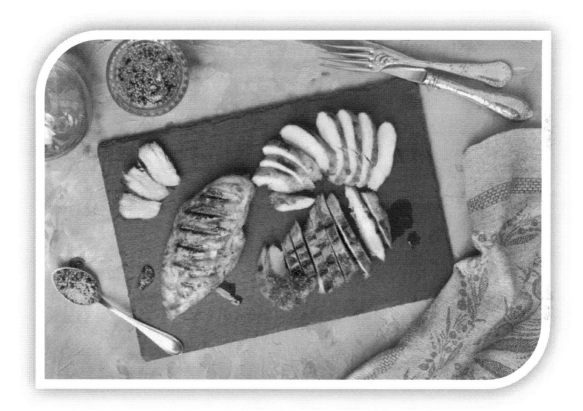

STEP 5: KEEP HYDRATED

When you're reducing your carb intake significantly you deplete your sugar stores, also know as glycogen. This stores three grams of water with each gram of glycogen. When you deplete them, the kidneys will excrete more water than usual, which will help you to lose an initial water weight at the beginning. However, there is a downside to this. You will lose electrolytes, and therefore dehydration is a common side effect. You should be drinking about a gallon of water a day to stay fit and healthy on the ketogenic diet. This means you'll need to keep water with you. Dehydration can cause keto flu like symptoms, headaches and even muscle cramps. Electrolytes are also critical to your success on the ketogenic diet, so make sure that you're getting enough magnesium, potassium and sodium. Always keep a water bottle with you.

STEP 6: DON'T EXPERIMENT YET

You don't want to experiment until the two-week mark. You must be in ketosis before your risk coming out of it, but if you experiment properly and keep an eye on what you're putting into your body, you should be able to stay in ketosis regardless. While a cheat day isn't possible on the ketogenic diet, experimental days are. Ones where you decide to snack more using fat bombs than you actually eat so that you can get the foods you love. Start with an easy and effective plan.

You'll want to make an easy shopping list that has ingredients that can be used more than once so you save money and time. Only add one thing at a time if you're having trouble with weight loss. For example, when you get started with ketosis but want to meal prep as well, don't do it too much. Start by just meal prepping your breakfast. This will save you time, and you know exactly what you're eating every morning. If you know how many net carbs you've consumed in the morning, you know how many you have left for the day. If you want to add in a day where you get dessert, don't add it on the day that you are going out with friends.

TIP 7: TRACK YOUR GOALS

A lot of people have a hard time getting into ketosis, and continuing to struggle without monitoring their progress is one of the biggest mistakes that can be made. This is where your journal comes in handy once again. When you first start ketosis, you will lose some water weight, but keep your goal light. Your first goal should be getting past the keto flu. Give yourself two full weeks, and expect minimal weight loss at best. You can then expect to lose roughly five pounds in a week once you're in ketosis, but it will mainly be water weight. When you have hit the five-pound mark, look at what you're eating. Keeping a food journal will help with this as well. After that, see where you can cut back or add in exercise. Every time you meet a goal, set another one. Try not to set your goals too far in advance. If you try to set your goals too far ahead, you're more likely to fall short of them.

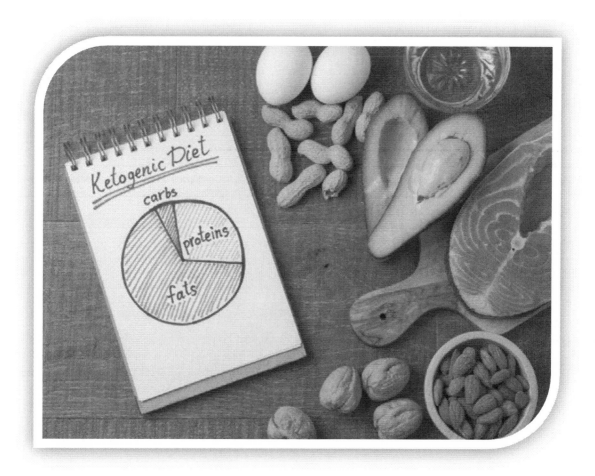

STEP 8: WORK IN SOME EXERCISE

It's important to add exercise into any diet, including the ketogenic diet. While you don't need to exercise too hard, it'll help you to tone up and lose weight in a healthy way. You need to be able to take at least twenty minutes each and every day. Of course, if you aren't used to exercising, you'll need to slowly add exercise in. while it's best to exercise for twenty to thirty minutes consecutively, you can break this into two ten-minute intervals to start with. So, going on the idea that you do not currently exercise, start by getting up and going on a ten minute walk every morning and every evening for three days.

After three days, start power walking for two fifteen intervals each day. Getting your heart pumping with this light cardio can be essential to your weight loss and health goals. After two more days of this, try jogging lightly. After two days of this go back to speed walking. Pulsing yourself too hard will make it difficult to continue. Now, once you feel more comfortable, you need to try to run to up your cardio even more.

Once you start to run and it becomes easy, you'll want to have a full running session once a day even if just for twenty minutes in the evening or morning, but you'll want to try to add something else in as well. While you don't need to add more time in per day, you'll want to vary your exercise. Try adding in some leg lifts, yoga, or even crunches once a week, and continue to add onto your regime from there. Now that you've gotten the hang of it, it'll make it easier to continue your diet and reach the weight loss goals that you've set for yourself.

STEP 9: TAKE TIME TO CHANGE YOUR MIND

Your mindset is more powerful than you think. If you go into the ketogenic diet thinking that it's going to be hard, then you're going to make it hard on yourself. Not everything will fall into place the moment you start thinking it will, but when you have set up goals that you're meeting and exercise daily, you just need to concentrate on keeping a positive attitude each and every day. You can do this by having a mantra as well as reminding yourself of all the goals that you've met thus far. Below you'll find a few mantras that you can use in the morning.

- I am going to stay in ketosis today.
- I am going to stick to my diet and be successful.
- I have come very far, and I will continue to reach my goals.
- I am happy with the progress that I have made thus far.

Saying these to yourself at least three times in front of the mirror in the morning will help you to stay in the correct mindset. Of course, you need mantras and reassurance when you make a mistake too, so try using some of the following.

- I am not my failures. I will get back into ketosis.

- I am able to get back on track and have not erased my goals.

- I am going to move forward and stick to the diet.

Just saying these out loud can help you to redirect your mindset so that you can get back to the ketogenic diet without beating yourself up over your mistakes. Mistakes will not make or break the ketogenic diet for you even if it may break your ketosis. You can always get back into ketosis.

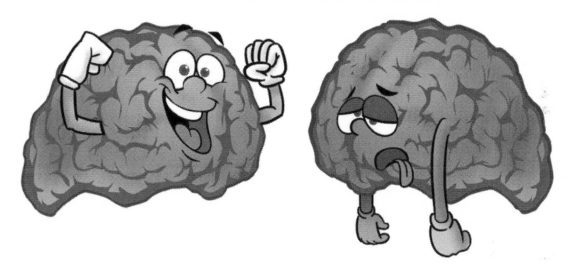

STEP 10: MAKE TIME FOR REWARDS

You'll need to make time for rewards as well. Don't ever reward yourself in a way that will break your ketosis. However, small rewards will keep you motivated for going forward, so take a moment to plan some out. Is there something you -really- like? Maybe it isn't ketogenic friendly, but usually you can work it in there if you're careful enough with the rest of your schedule. If you can, you can also look up a ketogenic version of it to reward yourself with when you reach a certain goal.

Maybe you really like cheese cake, but not all cheesecake is ketogenic friendly. Instead, look for a ketogenic friendly version. You can do this for just about anything, including espresso drinks, take out, and just about any food you can think of. It's best to start without sweets on a daily basis, so a dessert can also be a good addition to your ketogenic diet as a reward. Some possible rewards can be found below.

- Your favorite meal at a restaurant served in a ketogenic style.

- A sugar free beverage that you can't usually get due to the empty calories.

- One day where you skip exercise.

- Going to a favorite place, but remember to pack a ketogenic lunch!

Now that you have some reward ideas, try to make a reward tier. You should always reward yourself at least once a week if you haven't fallen off of the ketogenic wagon. This will help you to stay motivated to stay on track.

BREAKFAST
RECIPES

BRUSSEL & BACON HASH

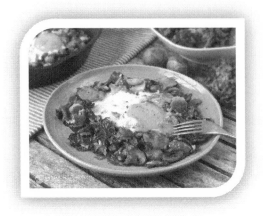

Serves: 3
Time: 25 Minutes
Calories: 220
Protein: 17 Grams
Fat: 13 Grams
Net Carbs: 8 Grams

Ingredients:

- **12 Ounces Brussel Sprouts, Sliced**
- **2 Cloves Garlic, Minced**
- **2 Shallots, Minced**
- **2 Ounces Bacon**
- **3 Eggs**
- **1 ℔ Tablespoons Apple Cider Vinegar**
- **Sea Salt & Black Pepper to Taste**

Directions:

1. Cook your bacon in a skillet using medium heat, and then place it to the side.
2. Use the drippings to cook your shallots and garlic for half a minute before adding in your Brussel sprouts. Add in the vinegar, and combine well. Cook for five minutes, but stir often so that it doesn't burn.
3. Add in the bacon again, and stir. Cook for another three minutes and then make a hole in the skillet. Add in your eggs, and scramble.

MUSHROOM OMELET

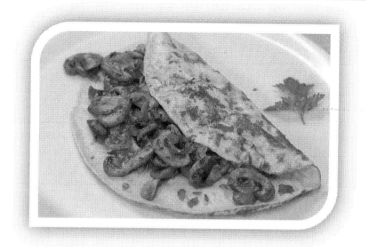

Serves: 4
Time: 30 Minutes
Calories: 109
Protein: 0.9 Grams
Fat: 9.6 Grams
Carbs: 6.2 Grams

Ingredients:

- 3 Eggs
- 1 Ounce Cheddar Cheese, Shredded
- 1 Ounce Butter
- 3 Mushrooms
- × Yellow Onion, Diced
- Sea Salt & Black Pepper to Taste

Directions:

1. Start by beating your eggs with salt and pepper, and then get out a frying pan. Melt the butter, and then pour in your egg mixture. Top with mushrooms, egg and cheese, flipping the egg over the filling. Cook for one minute per side.
2. Serve warm.

GREEK BREAKFAST BAKE

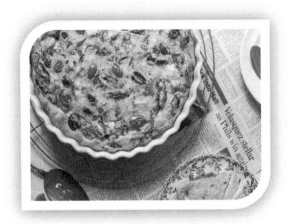

Serves: 10
Time: 30 Minutes
Calories: 139
Protein: 10.9 Grams
Fat: 10.1 Grams
Net Carbs: 2.3 Grams

Ingredients:

- 12 Eggs
- 1 Cup Kale, Chopped
- × Cup Sun Dried Tomatoes
- ℔ Teaspoon Oregano
- ℔ Cup Feta
- Sea Salt & Black Pepper to Taste

Directions:

1. Start by heating your oven to 350, and then whisk your eggs together with remaining ingredients.
2. Line a baking pan with parchment paper.
3. Pour it in, and bake for twenty-five minutes. Allow it to rest for five minutes before slicing to serve.

SARDINE & EGG DELIGHT

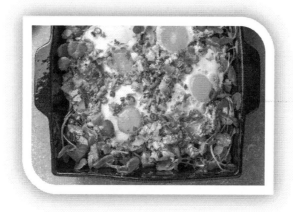

Serves: 2
Time: 10 Minutes
Calories: 250
Protein: 26 Grams
Fat: 13 Grams
Carbs: 2 Grams

Ingredients:

- 1 Can Sardines
- ⅕ Can Smoked Oysters
- 1 Tablespoon Oil
- Broccoli
- 2 Eggs

Directions:

1. Start by heating up a pan and pouring in your oil.
2. Add in your eggs, cooking for a minute.
3. Add in your broccoli and sardine, and then add in your smoked oysters. Stir well. Cook for four minutes.
4. Serve when heated all the way through and your eggs are set.

CHIA SEED PARFAIT

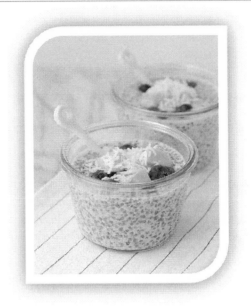

Serves: 3
Time: 20 Minutes
Calories: 160
Protein: 6 Grams
Fat: 10 Grams
Carbs: 4 Grams

Ingredients:

- × Teaspoon Cinnamon, Divided
- 6 Teaspoons Almond, Sliced& Divided
- 1 Cup Yogurt, Full Fat
- 2 Tablespoons Chia Seeds
- × Cup Almond Milk, Unsweetened

Directions:

1. Get out a medium bowl and mix your chia seeds, yogurt and almond milk in, and then get out a glass. Pour in a third of the mixture and then add in two teaspoons of almonds, and then a little cinnamon. repeat with the remaining ingredients.
2. Refrigerate for ten minutes, and then serve chilled.

COCONUT FLOUR WAFFLES

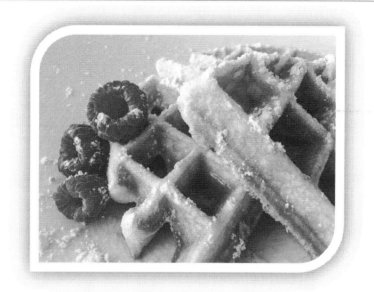

Serves: 4
Time: 10 Minutes
Calories: 366
Protein: 17.5 Grams
Fat: 25.8 Grams
Carbs: 4.25 Grams

Ingredients:

- 6 Eggs

- × Cup Coconut Oil

- 1 Teaspoon Cane Sugar, Raw

- ℔ Cup Coconut Flour, Sifted

- ℔ Teaspoon Baking Powder

- ℔ Teaspoon Sea Salt, Fine

Directions:

1. Whisk in your coconut oil and eggs until combined.

2. Get out a different bowl and mix your cane sugar, salt, baking powder and flour.

3. Mix it with the egg mixture, making sure it's beat smooth.

4. Allow the mixture to rest for ten minutes, and during this time it will rise some.

5. Get out a waffle maker, and preheat it. Make sure to lightly grease it with oil, and then cook like you normally would. It will need divided into four equal portions, and serve warm.

CREAM CHEESE & AVOCADO SCRAMBLE

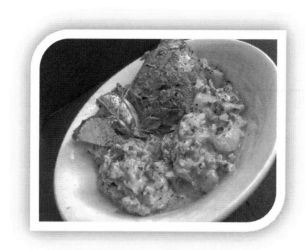

Serves: 4
Time: 15 Minutes
Calories: 444
Protein: 18 Grams
Fat: 38 Grams
Net Carbs: 3 Grams

Ingredients:

- 8 Eggs, Large

- 2 Tablespoons Heavy Cream

- Sea Salt & Black Pepper to Taste

- 2 Tablespoons Butter, Salted

- × Cup Cream Cheese

- ⅕ Cup Cheddar Cheese, Shredded

- 2 Avocados, Sliced

Directions:

1. Start by getting out a bowl and whisk your salt, pepper, cream and eggs

together until smooth.

2. Get out a skillet and melt your butter over medium heat. Add in the egg mix, and stir while cooking for four minutes. Your eggs should be halfway cooked.

3. Add in your cheese and cream cheese. Stir gently, and serve topped with avocado.

EASY ENGLISH BREAKFAST

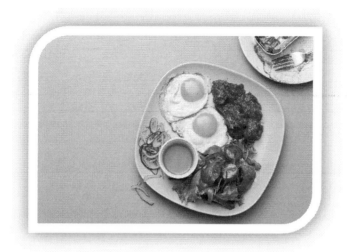

Serves: 4
Time: 25 Minutes
Calories: 404
Protein: 17 Grams
Fat: 34 Grams
Net Carbs: 4 Grams

Ingredients:

- 4 Eggs, Large

- 8 Bacon Slices, Uncured

- 2 Cups Mushrooms, Sliced

- 4 Sausage Links

- 2 Avocados, Sliced

- Sea Salt & Black Pepper to Taste

Directions:

1. Get out a skillet and scramble your eggs before placing them to the side. You can also fry them if you like.

2. Use the same skillet and cook your bacon and sausage until browned. It should take roughly ten minutes, and then line a plate with paper towels. Lay them on it to drain.

3. Add your sliced mushrooms in and then cook in the rendered bacon and sausage fat. Cook for five to six minutes. They should be softened and browned, but you'll need to stir constantly to keep from sticking.

4. Serve on a plate with avocado, and season with salt and pepper.

CHEESY EGG & AVOCADO BOATS

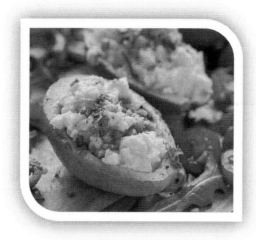

Serves: 4
Time: 25 Minutes
Calories: 324
Protein: 10.8 Grams
Fats: 28.5 Grams
Net Carbs: 6 Grams

Ingredients:

- 2 Eggs
- 1 Avocado, Halved
- 1/8 Teaspoon Black Pepper
- 1/8 Teaspoon Sea Salt, Fine
- 4 Tablespoons Colby Cheese, Shredded

Directions:

1. Start by heating your oven to 475, and then take the stone from your avocado. Scoop some of the flesh out, placing the flesh into a ramekin. Crack and egg into each avocado, and then sprinkle on your cheese. Season with salt and pepper, and then heat up the oven.
2. Add the avocado to your oven, making sure not to tip it. Use a baking sheet.
3. Bake for twenty minutes, and serve hot.

ASPARAGUS & EGG BAKE

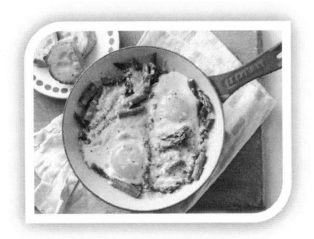

Serves: 4
Time: 25 Minutes
Calories: 370
Protein: 23 Grams
Fat: 27 Grams
Net Carbs: 3 Grams

Ingredients:

- 12 Bacon Slices, Uncured

- 18 Asparagus Spears, Trimmed

- 8 Eggs, Large

- 1 Avocado, Sliced

- Sea Salt & Black Pepper to Taste

Directions:

1. Start by heating the oven to 425, and then get out a cast iron skillet.

2. Place the skillet over medium heat to cook your bacon, and turn with tons every few minutes to ensure that it doesn't stick or burn. Don't cook it fully, but it should be mostly cooked.

3. Line a plate with paper towels, and then transfer the bacon onto it.

4. Discard all but three tablespoons of the bacon fat, and keep that in the pan. Add in your asparagus, seasoning with salt and pepper. Make sure they're well coated in the fat.

5. Bake for eight minutes in the oven. Your asparagus should soften, and then remove them from the oven. Turn with tons, and then add in your bacon. Cracked in the eggs, and then bake in the oven for seven more minutes. Your eggs should be done all the way through.

6. Serve with avocado slices.

LUNCH
RECIPES

LASAGNA STUFFED MUSHROOMS

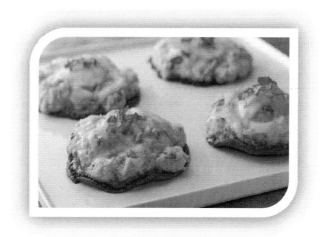

Serves: 4
Time: 30 Minutes
Calories: 261
Protein: 21 Grams
Fat: 16 Grams
Net Carbs: 11 Grams

Ingredients:

- 2 Tablespoons Olive Oil

- 1 ⅓ Cups Light Ricotta

- 1 Cup Marinara Sauce

- 4 Portobello Mushrooms, Large

- 1 Egg

- 1 ⅓ Cup Spinach, Chopped

- ⅓ Cup Basil, Fresh & Chopped

- 1 Cup Mozzarella, Shredded

- Pinch Sea Salt

Directions:

1. Start by heating your oven to 400, and then get out a baking sheet. Line it with parchment paper, and clean your mushrooms. Remove the gills and stem before washing them. Layer the mushrooms with olive oil, and add in × cup of marinara into each cap.

2. Add in the spinach, basil, egg, ricotta and salt. Toss well, and the divide it between all four mushrooms.

3. Top with mozzarella, and bake for twenty minutes. Serve warm.

PORK BELLY SALAD

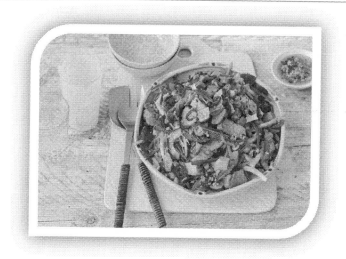

Serves: 4
Time: 15 Minutes
Calories: 152
Protein: 8.5 Grams
Fat: 10 Grams
Net Carbs: 6 Grams

Ingredients:

- 1 Head Iceberg Lettuce, Quartered
- 12 Ounces Pork Belly, Cooked Until Crisp & Chopped
- × Cup Blue Cheese Crumbles
- 12 Grape Tomatoes, Halved
- 2 Tablespoons Red Onion, Chopped

Directions:

1. Put each wedge on a plate and then top with remaining ingredients. Serve chilled or room temperature.

EASY TACO SALAD

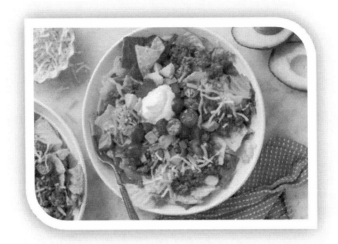

Serves: 6
Time: 15 Minutes
Calories: 467
Protein: 23 Grams
Fat: 36 Grams
Net Carbs: 8 Grams

Ingredients:

Salad:

- 1 lb. Ground Beef, Cooked

- 6 Cups Romain Lettuce, Chopped

- 1 Tomato, Diced

- 1 Cup Cheddar Cheese, Shredded

Topping:

- 1 Avocado, Sliced

- ⅓ Cup Sour Cream

- ⅓ Cup Salsa, Low Carb

- 1 Tablespoon Lime Juice, Fresh

- Sea Salt & Black Pepper to Taste

- Cilantro Leaves, Fresh & Chopped for Serving

- 1 Cup Ranch Dressing, Dairy Free

Directions:

2. Start by getting out a bowl and toss your meat, tomato, cheese and lettuce.

3. Divide the salad among the bowl and arrange your toppings before serving.

TUNA SALAD WRAPS

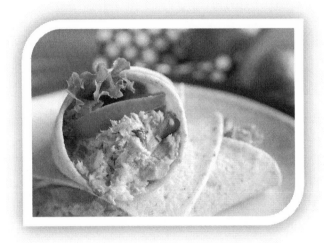

Serves: 2
Time: 15 Minutes
Calories: 506
Protein: 34 Grams
Fat: 36 Grams
Net Carbs: 6 Grams

Ingredients:

- 2 Cans Tuna, 12 Ounces Each & Drained

- Red Onion, Diced

- 1 Tomato, Diced

- 1 Tablespoon Lime Juice, Fresh

- × Cup Mayonnaise

- 1 Tablespoon Mustard

- 1 Tablespoon Celery Seed

- 1 Avocado, Sliced

- Romaine Lettuce Leaves for Serving

- **Sea Salt & Black Pepper to Taste**

Directions:

1. Start by combining all ingredients together except for your avocado and lettuce leaves.

2. Spoon the mixture onto your lettuce leaves and top with avocado before serving wrapped.

CRAB AVOCADO BOATS

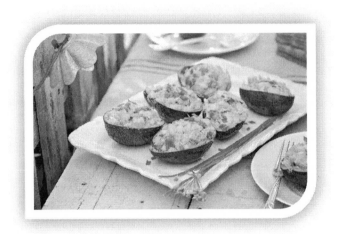

Serves: 4
Time: 15 Minutes
Calories: 350
Protein: 14 Grams
Fat: 29 Grams
Net Carbs: 3 Grams

Ingredients:

- 2 Avocados, Halved

- 1 Cup Celery, Chopped

- 12 Ounces Crab Meat

- 3 Scallions, Diced

- 6 Tablespoons Mayonnaise

- 1 Lemon, Juiced

- Lemon Wedges to Garnish

- 1 Teaspoon Paprika

- Sea Salt & Black Pepper to Taste

Directions:

1. Start by scooping the flesh from the avocado, but leave a thin layer attached. Dice the flesh into small pieces before placing it in ab owl.

2. Add all your ingredients except for your lemon wedges, and mix well.

3. Arrange this mixture into your avocado shells, and serve garnished with lemon wedges.

BLT KETO WRAPS

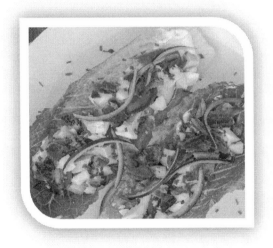

Serves: 2
Time: 10 Minutes
Calories: 585
Protein: 13 Grams
Fat: 54 Grams
Net Carbs: 8 Grams

Ingredients:

- 2 Tablespoons Mayonnaise
- 8 Romaine Lettuce Leaves
- Pinch Sea Salt
- × Teaspoon Black Pepper
- 6 Pieces Bacon, Cooked
- 1 Tomato, Diced
- 1 Avocado, Chopped

Directions:

1. Start by spooning the mayonnaise over four lettuce leaves. Season with salt and pepper, and then distribute your tomato, avocado, bacon and tomato amount the four leaves. Top with remaining leaves before serving.

SLOPPY JOE WRAPS

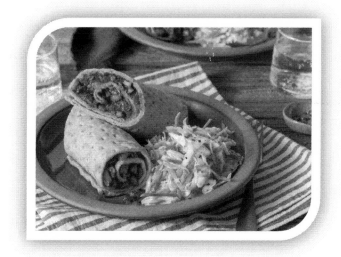

Serves: 4
Time: 30 Minutes
Calories: 272
Protein: 24 Grams
Fat: 18 Grams
Net Carbs: 4 Grams

Ingredients:

- 1 Tablespoon Olive Oil

- 1 Yellow Onion, Chopped

- 1 Green Bell Pepper, Chopped

- 1 lb. Ground Beef

- ⅓ Cup Ketchup, Sugar Free

- 1 Teaspoon Garlic Powder

- 1 Teaspoon Mustard

- 1 Tablespoon Worcestershire Sauce

- 1 Tablespoon Sugar Substitute

- Sea Salt & Black Pepper to Taste

- Lettuce Leaves for Serving

Directions:

1. Get out a skillet and place it over medium heat to heat up your olive oil. Add in your onion and pepper, and stir frequently. Cook for six minutes. They should be tender. Add in your ground beef, and brown for ten minutes. Make sure to break it up.

2. Stir in your garlic powder, mustard, Worcestershire sauce, ketchup, salt, pepper and sweetener. Bring it all to a boil, and then turn the heat to low. Let it simmer for ten minutes, and serve on lettuce leaves.

KETO BACON CHEESEBURGERS

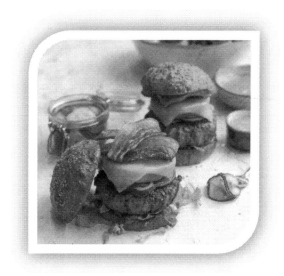

Serves: 4
Time: 30 Minutes
Calories: 560
Protein: 35 Grams
Fat: 41 Grams
Net Carbs: 7 Grams

Ingredients:

- 1 lb. Ground Beef

- Sea Salt & Black Pepper to Taste

- 8 Bacon Slices, Uncured

- 8 Slices Cheddar Cheese

- Iceberg Lettuce to Serve

- × Cup Mayonnaise

- × Cup Ketchup, Sugar Free

- 2 Tomatoes, Sliced

- 1 Avocado, Sliced

Directions:

1. Season your ground beef using salt and pepper, and then form the meat into four patties.

2. Get out a skillet and place it over medium heat, and cook until the bacon reaches the desired crisp. It should take eight to ten minutes, and then place it on a plate lined with paper towels to drain. Remove half of your bacon grease, but use the rest to cook the burgers.

3. Return the skillet to your stovetop to cook the patties for five minutes per side.

4. Add two pieces of cheese before serving warm on the lettuce leaves with ketchup and mayonnaise. Top with avocados, bacon and tomatoes before wrapping up to serve.

CHICHARRONS NACHOS

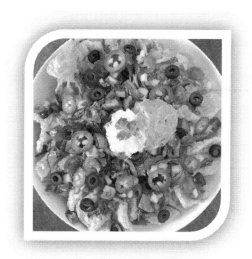

Serves: 4
Time: 15 Minutes
Calories: 515
Protein: 30 Grams
Fat: 41 Grams
Net Carbs: 5 Grams

Ingredients:

- 16 Ounce Bag Chicharrons

- ½lb. Ground Beef, Cooked

- 2 Cups Cheddar Cheese, Shredded

- 6 Ounces Black Olives, Canned, Drained & Sliced

- 2 Tomatoes, Diced

- ½ Cup Sour Cream

- 1 Avocado, Sliced

- Jalapeno Pepper, Sliced to Serve

Directions:

1. Start by turning the broiler on in your oven, and then get out a baking pan. Line it with foil, and spread the pork rinds out in a single layer. Top with cheese and meat, and broil for five minutes. Make sure it doesn't burn.

2. Top with tomatoes, avocado, sour cream, peppers and avocado before serving.

CHEESESTEAK ROLLUPS

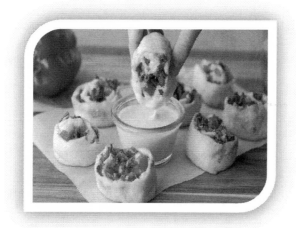

Serves: 4
Time: 30 Minutes
Calories: 475
Protein: 33 Grams
Fat: 35 Grams
Net Carbs: 5 Grams

Ingredients:

- 1 lb. Sirloin Tip Steak

- Sea Salt & Black Pepper to Taste

- 6 Slices Provolone Cheese

- 1 Cup mushrooms, Chopped

- 1 Yellow Onion, Diced

- 1 Green Bell Pepper, Seeded & Diced

- × Cup Butter, Salted

Directions:

1. Start by pounding your steak down to × inch thickness before seasoning with salt and pepper.

2. Get out a skillet and add in your butter. Put it over medium heat, and then let your butter melt. Once it's melted add in your pepper, onion, and mushrooms, cook for six minutes, but stir frequently to avoid burning. Your vegetable should be tender.

3. Spread it over the prepared steak in an even layer before topping with the cheese slices.

4. Roll the steak into a pin wheel, and then secure with toothpicks. It's best to place them two inches apart, and cut between them.

5. Cook your pinwheels in your skillet for seven-minutes per side, and serve warm.

STUFFED AVOCADOS

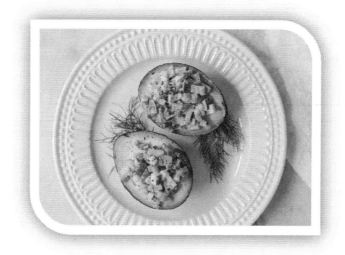

Serves: 4
Time: 20 Minutes
Calories: 390
Protein: 18 Grams
Fat: 32 Grams
Net Carbs: 3 Grams

Ingredients:

- Avocados, Halved

- 1 Tablespoon Lime Juice, Fresh

- 4 Ounces Cream Cheese, Room Temperature

- 1 Cup Shredded Chicken, Favored

- ½ Teaspoon Ground Cumin

- ½ Teaspoon Garlic Powder

- 1 Cup Colby Jack Cheese, Shredded

- Sea Salt & Black Pepper to Taste

Directions:

1. Start by heating your oven to 400, and then get out a baking sheet. Line it with foil, and scoop the flesh from your avocado. Make sure not to tear the shells, but set them aside. Put your flesh in a bowl.

2. In that bowl add in your remaining ingredients except for cheese and then scoop the mixture back into your avocados. Sprinkle with cheese, and bake for ten minutes. Serve warm.

KETO CHICKEN & BACON BURGERS

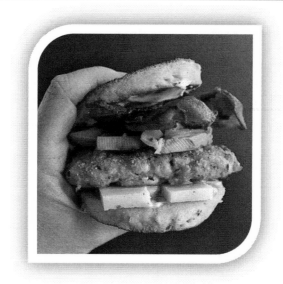

Serves: 4
Time: 30 Minutes
Calories: 435
Protein: 34 Grams
Fat: 31 Grams
Net Carbs: 2 Grams

Ingredients:

- 4 Chicken Breasts, Skin On & Boneless

- 8 Slices Bacon, Uncured

- 4 Slices Pepper Jack Cheese

- Sea Salt & Black Pepper to Taste

- × Cup Mayonnaise

- 8 Romain Lettuce Leaves

- 1 Avocado, Sliced

Directions:

1. Start by laying your bacon in a cold skillet before putting it over medium-

low. It should reach desired crispness, but may take up to eight minutes to cook. Transfer it to a plate that's been lined in paper towels to drain.

2. Eason your chicken using salt and pepper and cook in the bacon grease for ten minutes per side. It should be cooked all the way.

3. Layer two pieces of bacon with a slice of cheese and a chicken breast. Divide your mayonnaise among four lettuce leaves, and then put your chicken breast on each. Top with avocado and the remaining lettuce leaves. Serve warm.

KETO CHICKEN CLUB SANDWICHES

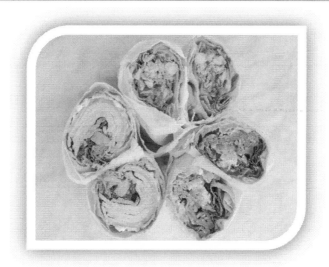

Serves: 4
Time: 35 Minutes
Calories: 405
Protein: 26 Grams
Fat: 29 Grams
Net Carbs: 5 Grams

Ingredients:

- 1 Tomato, Diced
- 1 Avocado, Sliced
- 2 Cups Salsa Shredded chicken
- 6 Slices Bacon, Cooked & Crumbled
- 4 Tablespoons Blue Cheese Crumbles
- Sea Salt & Black Pepper to taste
- ⅓ Cup Ranch Dressing, Dairy Free
- 8 Romain Lettuce Leaves for Serving

Directions:

1. Start by diving everything between your lettuce leaves, and drizzle with ranch before wrapping to serve. Serve chilled or room temperature.

CILANTRO CHICKEN FAJITAS

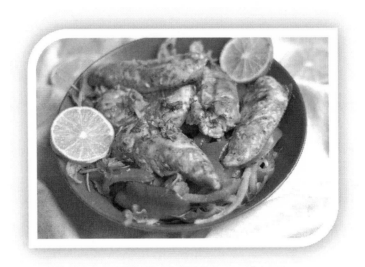

Serves: 4
Time: 30 Minutes
Calories: 522
Protein: 35 Grams
Fat: 37 Grams
Net Carbs: 10 Grams

Ingredients:

- 1/3 Cup Cilantro Leaves, Fresh & Chopped
- 1 lb. Chicken Breasts, Boneless, Skinless & Sliced
- 3 Tablespoons Olive Oil, Divided
- 1 Teaspoon Ground Cumin
- 1 Clove Garlic, Minced
- 1 Teaspoon Sea Salt + More as Needed
- 2 Bell Peppers, Seeded & Sliced Thin
- 1 Yellow Onion, Sliced Thin
- Black Pepper to Taste

To Serve:

- 1 Cup Sour Cream
- 1 Avocado, Sliced
- 1 Cup Cheddar Cheese, Shredded

Directions:

2. Combine your chicken breast once sliced, a tablespoon of oil, cumin, garlic, salt and cilantro together. Toss and make sure that your chicken is well coated.

3. Get out a skillet and place it over heat with tablespoon of oil, and then cook your bell peppers and onion. Stir so it doesn't burn, and cook for seven minutes. It should be softening and lightly browned. Line a plat with paper towels, and then place them on the plate to drain away any excess grease.

4. Use the same skillet to cook your chicken, and make sure it's cooked all the way through while stirring occasionally to avoid sticking. Cook for twelve minutes.

5. Return your bell pepper and onion to the skillet to heat up until they begin to sizzle.

6. Season with salt and pepper, and serve topped with avocado slices, cheese and sour cream.

TWISTED CHICKEN NUGGETS

Serves: 6
Time: 20 Minutes
Calories: 150
Protein: 15 Grams
Fat: 18 Grams
Net Carbs: 1.8 Grams

Ingredients:

- 2 Cups Chicken, Cooked

- 8 Ounces Cream Cheese

- cup Almond Flour

- 1 Egg

- 1 Teaspoon Garlic Salt

Directions:

1. Get out an electric mixture and shred your chicken. Add in all remaining ingredients, and then flatten into nugget shapes on a greased baking pan.

2. Bake at 350 for thirteen minutes. They should turn golden, and enjoy warm.

DINNER
RECIPES

BACON BURGER CASSEROLE

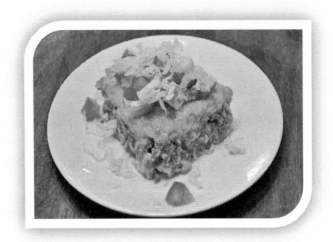

Serves: 10
Time: 30 Minutes
Calories: 613
Protein: 33 Grams
Fat: 51 Grams
Net Carbs: 3 Grams

Ingredients:

- Beef Layer:

- 1 ℔ lbs. Ground Beef

- 1 Clove Garlic, Crushed

- 1 Onion, Sliced

- 3 Slices Bacon, Diced

- Sea Salt & Black Pepper to Taste

- 2.25 Ounces Cream Cheese

Cheese Sauce:

- 3 Eggs

- 3.5 Ounces Cheddar Cheese, Shredded

- 125 mL Heavy Cream

- 2 Sliced Pickles

- 2 Tablespoons Mustard

- 1.75 Ounces Pepper Jack, Shredded & Reserved

Directions:

1. Start by cooking your bacon, and then put it to the side.

2. Cook your garlic, beef, and onion in the drippings until the beef is thoroughly cooked. Season with salt and pepper before adding in your cream cheese.

3. Pour this mixture into the baking dish, and sprinkle with bacon bits.

4. Make your cheese sauce next. Combine your cheese, salt, pepper, eggs, and mustard, and mix well. Pour this over the bacon mixture, and then add your pickles. Coat with the pepper jack.

5. Bake at 350 for fifteen minutes, and serve warm.

STEAK SALAD

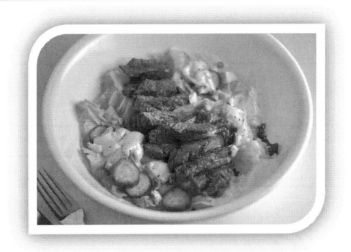

Serves: 4
Time: 20 Minutes
Calories: 541
Protein: 24 Grams
Fat: 46 Grams
Net Carbs: 3 Grams

Ingredients:

- Cup + 2 Tablespoons Olive Oil, Divided

- 12 Ounces Flank Steak

- Sea Salt & Black Pepper to Taste

- 6 Cups Spinach, Fresh

- 2 Avocados, Cubed

- 4 Ounces Feta Cheese, Crumbled

- 1 Lemon, Juiced

Directions:

1. Start by setting the broiler to high, and then rub two tablespoons of olive

oil over the steak.

2. Place the steak on a broiler pan, and broil for four minutes per side.

3. Transfer to a cutting board and allow it to rest for ten minutes.

4. While it's resting toss your avocado, spinach and feta cheese together. Add in the remaining olive oil, lemon juice, and salt and pepper. Toss until well combined, and divide between four bowls.

5. Top with sliced flank steak.

SALMON & ASPARAGUS DINNER

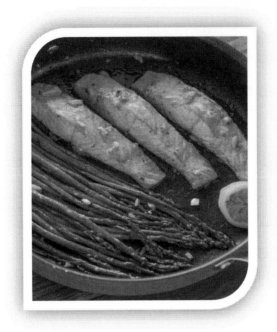

Serves: 4
Time: 25 Minutes
Calories: 475
Protein: 36 Grams
Fat: 35 Grams
Net Carbs: 4 Grams

Ingredients:

- 4 Salmon Fillets, 6 Ounces Each

- 1 Lemon, Juiced

- 1 Teaspoon Garlic Salt, Divided

- 5 Tablespoons Olive Oil, Divided

- 1 lb. Asparagus, Trimmed

- Sea Salt & Black Pepper to Taste

Directions:

1. Start by putting your oven on broil and get out a baking pan. Line it with foil.

2. Rub your fillets down with olive oil and garlic salt. Arrange them on the pan, and squeeze the lemon juice on top.

3. Place your asparagus around it, drizzling with olive oil, and make sure it's well coated before seasoning with salt and pepper.

4. Cook for ten to twelve minutes. Your salmon should flake easily.

CREAMY LEMON TILAPIA BAKE

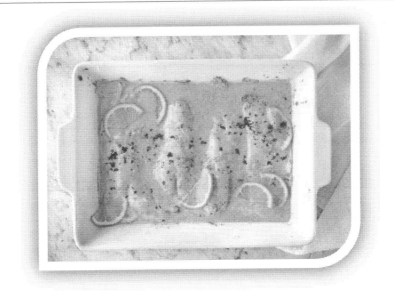

Serves: 4
Time: 25 Minutes
Calories: 369
Protein: 35 Grams
Fat: 25 Grams
Net Carbs: 2 Grams

Ingredients:

- 4 Tilapia Fillets, 6 Ounces Each

- 1 Teaspoon Garlic Powder

- Sea Salt & Black Pepper to Taste

- × Cup Butter, Salted & Room Temperature

- × Cup Heavy Cream

- × Cup Cream Cheese, Room Temperature

- 1 Tablespoon Mustard

- 2 Tablespoons Lemon Juice, Fresh

Directions:

1. Start by heating the oven to 400.

2. Get out a nine by thirteen-inch baking dish, and put your fillets in a single layer. Season with salt, pepper and garlic powder.

3. Get out a bowl and combine your butter, cream cheese, mustard, cream, and lemon juice. Microwave for thirty seconds, and stir in-between. It should be microwaved for two minutes total.

4. Pour this over the fish and bake for fifteen minutes. The fish should flake and be cooked all the way through.

KETO SHRIMP ALFREDO

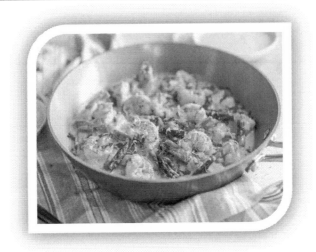

Serves: 3
Time: 25 Minutes
Calories: 558
Protein: 39 Grams
Fat: 37 Grams
Net Carbs: 14 Grams

Ingredients:

- 3 Tablespoons Butter, Salted & Divided

- 1 lb. Shrimp, Large, Peeled & Deveined

- Sea Salt & Black Pepper to Taste

- 4 Zucchini, Spiralized,

- 1 Cup Alfredo Sauce

- Cup Parmesan Cheese, Grated

Directions:

1. Start by getting out a large skillet and then cook a tablespoon of butter over medium heat, and then add int eh shrimp. Season with salt and pepper.

2. Cook your shrimp for four to six minutes, and make sure they're cooked on each side. Stir to keep them from sticking, and then line a plate with paper towels. Place your shrimp on it to drain.

3. Get out a skillet and melt the remaining butter. Add in your zucchini noodles and to with the remaining butter sauté for five minutes, and then add in the alfredo sauce and shrimp. Warm for five minutes, and serve immediately. Top with parmesan.

ONE PAN SHRIMP FAJITAS

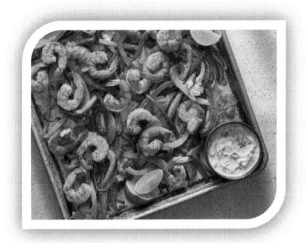

Serves: 4
Time: 20 Minutes
Calories: 635
Protein: 54 Grams
Fat: 41 Grams
Net Carbs: 10 Grams

Ingredients:

- 2 lbs. Shrimp, Large, Peeled & Deveined

- Olive Oil for Cooking

- 1 Green Bell Pepper, Seeded & Chopped

- 1 Red Bell Pepper, Seeded & Chopped

- 1 Red Onion, Chopped

- × Cup + 1 Tablespoon Olive Oil

- 1 Teaspoon Sea Salt

- 1 Teaspoon Black Pepper

- 1 Teaspoon Garlic Powder

- 1 Teaspoon Ground Cumin

- ⅓ Cup Sour Cream

- 1 Avocado, Sliced

- 1 Cup Colby Jack Cheese, Shredded

Directions:

1. Start by heating your oven to 400, and then get out a sheet pan. Line it with foil, and then get out a zipper top plastic bag. In that bag combine your bell peppers, onion, olive oil, salt, pepper, shrimp, cumin, lime juice, and garlic powder shake well until it's coated generously.

2. Pour this into your sheet pan, and then cook for ten minutes. Your shrimp should be cooked all the way.

3. Serve topped with sour cream, cheese and avocado slices.

CARAMELIZED RIBEYE DELIGHT

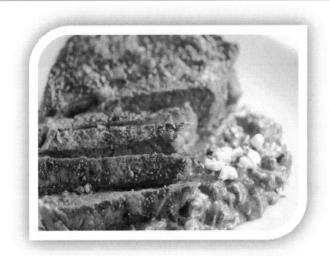

Serves: 2
Time: 30 Minutes
Calories: 519
Protein: 52 Grams
Fat: 31 Grams
Net Carbs: 5 Grams

Ingredients:

- 2 Ribeye Steaks, 6 Ounces Each

- Sea Salt & Black Pepper to Taste

- 1 Tablespoon Olive Oil

- 2 Tablespoons Ghee

- 1 Yellow Onion, Sliced

- 1 Cup Mushrooms, Sliced

Directions:

1. Pat the steaks down with a paper towel, and then rub hem down with olive oil. Season with salt and pepper and get out a skillet. Place it over medium heat to melt your butter.

2. Adding your onion, and stir frequently. Cook for four to five minutes. They should start to soften, and then add in your mushrooms. Cook until tender, which should take roughly five minutes more. Transfer to a plate lined with paper towels t drain.

3. Put the skillet over medium-high heat, and cook your steak for five minutes per side. Put the steak on a plate to rest for five more minutes.

4. Serve topped with your caramelized onion and mushrooms.

KETO BEEF STROGANOFF

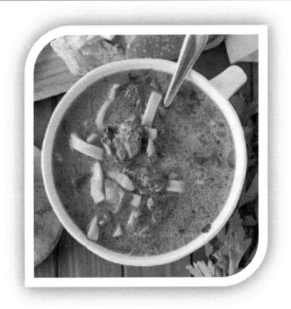

Serves: 4
Time: 25 Minutes
Calories: 369
Protein: 28 Grams
Fat: 25 Grams
Net Carbs: 7 Grams

Ingredients:

- 1 lb. Ground Beef

- 2 Cups Mushrooms, Sliced

- 1 Yellow Onion, Diced

- 1 Tablespoon Butter, Salted

- 3 Cloves Garlic, Minced

- 1 Cup Sour Cream

- 1 Cup Beef Broth

- × Teaspoon Xanthan Gum

- Sea Salt & Black Pepper to Taste

- Parsley, Fresh & Chopped to Garnish

- Grated Parmesan Cheese for Garnish

Directions:

1. Start by getting out a skillet and cook your beef over medium-high heat. Break it up, and cook until it's no longer pink. It should cook for ten minutes, and rain the fat away. Transfer it to a paper towel lined plate to finish draining.

2. Melt your butter and add in your mushrooms, garlic and onion. Cook while stirring frequently. Cook for about seven minutes.

3. Add in your browned beef, sour cream, xanthan gum, and broth. Stir well and cook for three to five minutes. The sauce should thicken. Serve garnished with cheese and parsley.

SIRLOIN STIR FRY & TOMATOES

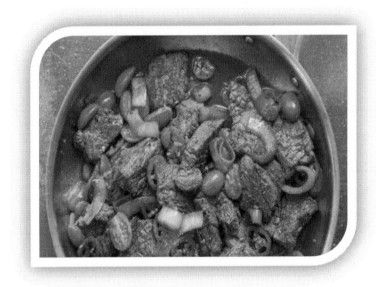

Serves: 2
Time: 20 Minutes
Calories: 437
Protein: 36 Grams
Fats: 29 Grams
Net Carbs: 6 Grams

Ingredients:

- 4 Cloves Garlic, Minced

- ℔ lb. Sirloin Steak, Cubed

- 4 Tablespoons Oregano, Fresh & Chopped

- 4 Ounces Cherry Tomatoes, Halved

- 3 Tablespoons Olive Oil

- Sea Salt & Black Pepper to Taste

Directions:

1. Start by heating your oil in a frying pan using medium heat, and then add in your steak. Cook until it browns, but you'll need to stir frequently to avoid burning.

2. Stir in your garlic for a minute. It should turn a golden brown. Season with salt and pepper, and then transfer to a plate.

3. Sprinkle with oregano and serve with cherry tomatoes.

WALNUT & ROSEMARY PORK LOIN

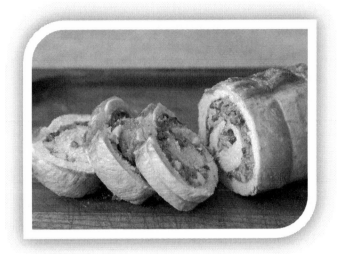

Serves: 4
Time: 30 Minutes
Calories: 535
Protein: 35 Grams
Fats: 42 Grams
Net Carbs: 5 Grams

Ingredients:

- 1 lb. Pork Loin

- 5 Tablespoons Rosemary, Fresh & Chopped

- 2 Ounces Walnuts, Chopped

- 8 Tablespoons Sour Cream

- 1/4 Cup Olive Oil

- Sea Salt & Black Pepper to Taste

Directions:

1. Start by heating the oven to 375.

2. Mix in your salt, pepper, olive oil and rosemary into your pork lin. Make sure it's evenly coated.

3. Put it on a baking pan, and then cover with foil.

4. Bake for twenty-five minutes, and allow it to bake for five more minutes or until golden brown.

5. Let it sit for five minutes before slicing.

6. Top with sour cream and walnuts before serving warm.

TWISTED PESTO CASSEROLE

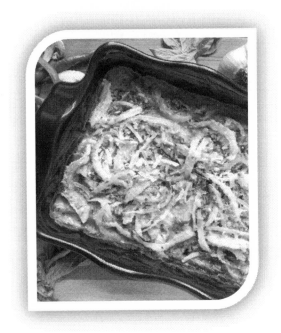

Serves: 8
Time: 30 Minutes
Calories: 451
Protein: 38 Grams
Fat: 30 Grams
Net Carbs: 3 Grams

Ingredients:

- 1/2 Cup Heavy Cream

- 8 Ounces Cream Cheese, Softened

- 1/4 Cup Pesto

- 8 Ounces Mozzarella, Shredded

- 8 Ounces Mozzarella, Cubed

- 2 lbs. Chicken Breasts, Cubed

Directions:

1. Start by preheating your oven to 400, and then get a casserole dish out. Spray it down with cooking spray, and then combine your pesto, cream cheese and heavy cream. Mix until a paste has formed, and then add in your cubed mozzarella and chicken.

2. Pour in your casserole dish, and then sprinkle with shredded mozzarella.

3. Bake for twenty-five minutes, and then serve warm or topped over zoodles.

CHEESY CHICKEN IN VODKA SAUCE

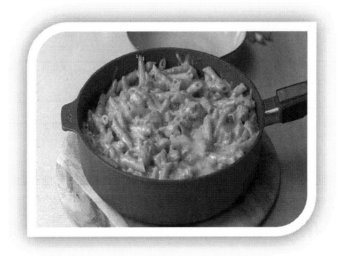

Serves: 8
Time: 30 Minutes
Calories: 236
Protein: 25.1 Grams
Fats: 13.2 Grams
Net Carbs: 4.7 Grams

Ingredients:

- **2 lbs. Chicken Breast, Cooked & Chunked**
- **1 1/2 Cups Vodka Sauce**
- **1/2 Cup Parmesan Cheese**
- **16 Ounces Fresh Mozzarella, Chunked**
- **Baby Spinach, Fresh**

Directions:

1. Start by heating your oven to 400, and then spray your casserole dish down. Add in your cooked chicken and top with cheese, mozzarella and vodka sauce.

2. Bake for twenty-five minutes. It should be bubbly. Serve topped with baby spinach. Your sauce should be hot enough to wilt it.

CHICKEN & RANCH CASSEROLE

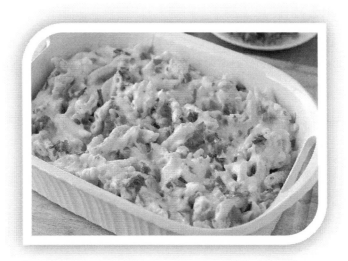

Serves: 6
Time: 30 Minutes
Calories: 521
Protein: 40 Grams
Fat: 37 Grams
Net Carbs: 6 Grams

Ingredients:

- 10 Slices Bacon, Cooked& Crumbled

- 4 Cups Seasoned Chicken, Shredded

- Salted Butter to Grease

- 16 Ounces Spinach, Frozen, Thawed & Drained

- 2 Cloves Garlic, Minced

- 1 Cup Ranch Dressing, Dairy Free

- 1/4 Cup Scallions, Sliced

- 1 Cup Mozzarella Cheese, Shredded & Divided

- 1 Cup Cheddar Cheese, Shredded & Divided

Directions:

1. Start by heating your oven to 375, and then get out a nine by thirteen-inch pan. Grease your pan with butter.

2. Get out a bowl and combine your ranch dressing, garlic, bacon, spinach, chicken, scallions, half a cup of both cheeses, and then mix well.

3. Pour into your baking dish and top with remaining cheeses.

4. Bake for twenty minutes. It should be bubbly and golden brown. Serve warm.

ITALIAN STUFFED CHICKEN

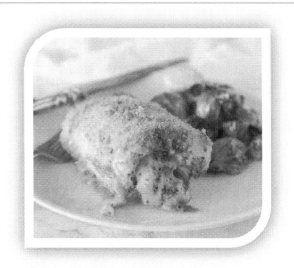

Serves: 4
Time: 25 Minutes
Calories: 465
Protein: 37 Grams
Fat: 34 Grams
Net Carbs: 2 Grams

Ingredients:

- 8 Basil Leaves, Large

- 1 Tomato, Sliced

- 8 Slices Mozzarella Cheese

- Sea Salt & Black Pepper to Taste

- 4 Chicken Breasts, Skin On & Boneless

- 1 Teaspoon Garlic Powder

- 3 Tablespoons Olive Oil, Divided

Directions:

1. Start by heating the oven to 350, and then get to your chicken breasts. Rub

olive oil on each one before seasoning with garlic, salt and pepper.

2. Cut a slit horizontally, but do not cut all the way through. You just need to create a pocket.

3. Layer your basil, tomato and mozzarella in the middle before closing the pocket by folding the chicken back over.

4. Get out a cast iron skillet and place it over medium heat. Heat up two tablespoons of oil, and then add your chicken breasts in with the skin side down. Cook for five minutes per side. Your skin should turn golden brown.

5. Transfer to the oven and bake for ten to twelve more minutes. Your chicken should be cooked all the way through. Serve warm.

TUNA TRUFFLE STEAKS

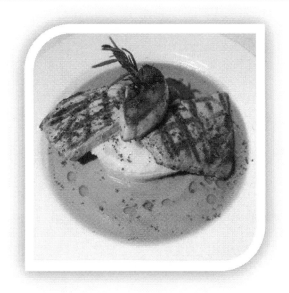

Serves: 3
Time: 15 Minutes
Calories: 380
Protein: 40 Grams
Fat: 23 Grams
Carbs: 1 Gram

Ingredients:

- 1 1/2 lbs. Tuna Steaks, Fresh
- 2 Tablespoons Truffle Oil
- 2 Tablespoons Oregano, Fresh & Chopped
- 3 Tablespoons Olive Oil

Directions:

1. Start by rubbing the truffle oil onto both sides of your tuna steaks evenly.
2. Place your olive oil in a frying pan, heating it up over high heat.
3. Add in the tuna steaks, cooking for four minutes per side.
4. Serve topped with fresh and chopped oregano.

SAGE RIBS & PEPPERS

Serves: 2
Time: 30 Minutes
Calories: 199
Protein: 31 Grams
Fats: 38 Grams
Net Carbs: 5 Grams

Ingredients:

- 1/2 lb. Pork Ribs
- 3 Tablespoons Butter
- 5 Tablespoons Sage, Fresh & Chopped
- 2 Bell Peppers, Seeded & Chopped
- Sea Salt & Black Pepper to Taste

Directions:

1. Start by heating your oven to 400 and then get out a baking pan. Grease it using butter.
2. Season the pork ribs using salt and pepper.
3. Heat up your remaining butter in a large frying pan, using medium heat, and fry the pork ribs to brown them. Put them on the grease baking pan, and sprinkle your chopped bell pepper and sage over it. Cover with foil.
4. Bake for twenty-five minutes, and then remove foil. Bake for five remaining minutes before serving warm.

SIDE DISH
RECIPES

ARTICHOKE DIP

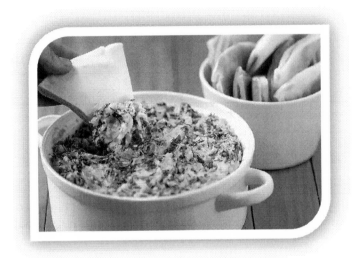

Serves: 6
Time: 10 Minutes
Calories: 475
Protein: 31 Grams
Fat: 36 Grams
Net Carbs: 6 Grams

Ingredients:

- 2 Tablespoons Olive Oil

- 1 lb. Goat Cheese

- 14 Ounces Artichoke Hearts, Canned & Drained

- 2 Teaspoons Lemon Juice

- 1 Clove Garlic, Minced

- 1 Tablespoon Parsley, Fresh & Chopped

- 1/2 Cup Parmesan Cheese, Grated

- 1 Tablespoon Chives, Fresh & Chopped

- 1/2 Tablespoon Basil, Fresh & Chopped

- Sea Salt & Black Pepper to Taste

Directions:

1. Start by blending everything together in a food processor before serving with vegetable chips.

CREAMED SPINACH

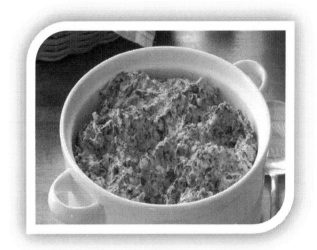

Serves: 4
Time: 15 Minutes
Calories: 387
Protein: 10 Grams
Fat: 37 Grams
Net Carbs: 4 Grams

Ingredients:

- 4 Tablespoons Butter, Salted & Divided

- 3 Cloves Garlic, Minced

- 20 Ounces Spinach, Frozen, Thawed, Drained & Chopped

- 2 Tablespoons Sour Cream

- 4 Ounces Cream Cheese

- 1/2 Cup Parmesan Cheese, Grated

- 1/2 Cup Heavy Cream

- Sea Salt & Black Pepper

1. Start by getting out a large skillet and melt two tablespoons of butter using medium heat. Cook your garlic for two minutes, stirring often so that it doesn't burn. Add in your spinach, and stir until all liquid has evaporated. This should take about five minutes.

2. Add in your heavy cream, sour cream, cream cheese, parmesan cheese, remaining two tablespoons of butter, and salt and pepper. Cook while stirring until it's all melted together. Cook for three minutes, and serve hot.

CAULIFLOWER & BROCCOLI MEDLEY

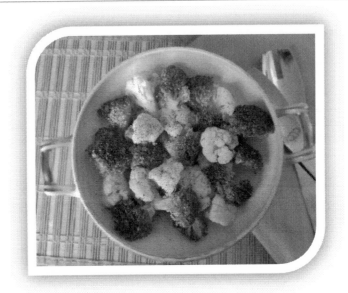

Serves: 4
Time: 30 Minutes
Calories: 221
Protein: 9 Grams
Fat: 19 Grams
Net Carbs: 2 Grams

Ingredients:

- 2 Cups Cauliflower Florets

- 2 Cups Broccoli Florets

- 1/4 Cup Olive Oil

- 2/3 Cup Parmesan Cheese, Grated

- 1 Teaspoon Garlic Powder

- 1 Teaspoon Onion Powder

- Sea Salt & Black Pepper to Taste

Directions:

1. Start by heating the oven to 400, and then line a baking sheet with foil.

2. Get out a zipper top bag and then toss your broccoli, cauliflower and olive oil together with your remaining half of your cheese. Add in your garlic, onion, salt and pepper, and shake until well coated.

3. Bake for about fifteen minutes. It might take twenty, but stir halfway through and make sure it doesn't burn. The edges should be browned.

4. Sprinkle over the remaining parmesan cheese, and top with more salt and pepper if desired. Serve warm.

BACON BRUSSEL SPROUTS

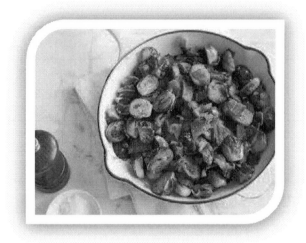

Serves: 4
Time: 30 Minutes
Calories: 512
Protein: 12 Grams
Fat: 49 Grams
Net Carbs: 6 Grams

Ingredients:

- 4 Cups Brussel Sprouts, Trimmed & Halved
- 1/4 Cup Olive Oil
- 2 Teaspoons Garlic Salt
- 12 Bacon Slices, Uncured & Chopped into 1 Inch Pieces

Directions:

1. Start by heating your oven to 400, and then get out a baking sheet. Line it with foil, and then get out a large bowl.
2. Mix your bacon, olive oil, garlic salt and sprouts together.
3. Spread it onto your pan in an even layer, and roast for a half hour. Turn once during this process, and then serve warm.

PROSCIUTTO ASPARAGUS

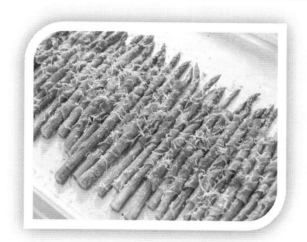

Serves: 4
Time: 20 Minutes
Calories: 222
Protein: 11 Grams
Fats: 19 Grams
Net Carbs: 1 Gram

Ingredients:

- 12 Asparagus Spears
- 5 Ounces Goat Cheese
- 2 Ounces Prosciutto, Sliced Thin
- 1/4 Teaspoon Black Pepper
- 2 Tablespoons Olive Oil

Directions:

1. Heat your oven to 450, and then put on the broiler function. Wash and trim your asparagus before slicing your cheese into twelve pieces, and then divide them into two.
2. Cut the slices of prosciutto lengthwise, and wrap around your asparagus with two cheese pieces.
3. Put them in a baking dish, and then sprinkle over your pepper. Drizzle with oil, and broil for fifteen minutes before serving.

KETO MAC & CHEESE

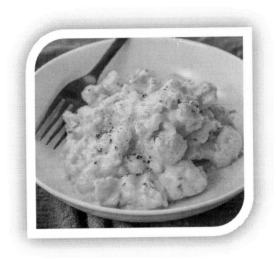

Serves: 2a
Time: 25 Minutes
Calories: 294
Protein: 11 Grams
Fat: 23 Grams
Net Carbs: 5 Grams

Ingredients:

- 1 Head Cauliflower, Chopped into Florets

- 2 Tablespoons Butter

- 1/4 Cup Heavy Cream

- 1/4 Cup Almond Milk, Unsweetened

- 1 Cup Cheddar Cheese, Shredded

- Sea Salt & Black Pepper to Taste

Directions:

1. Start by heating your oven to 450, and then get a baking sheet out. Line it

with foil, and then melt two tablespoons of butter and place it in a bowl. Toss in your florets before seasoning with salt and pepper.

2. Arrange the florets on your baking sheet, and cook for fifteen minutes.

3. Get out a heated pot and pour in your cheddar cheese, milk and heavy cream. Add in the remaining butter, and stir until all your cheese has melted.

4. Toss in your florets before serving, and make sure they're well coated.

CHEESY "RICE"

Serves: 4
Time: 25 Minutes
Calories: 297
Protein: 10 Grams
Fat: 25 Grams
Net Carbs: 7 Grams

Ingredients:

- 3 Tablespoons Butter, Salted

- 1 Yellow Onion, Diced

- 1/3 Cup Heavy Whipping Cream

- 4 Cups Cauliflower Rice

- 1 Teaspoon Garlic Powder

- 1 Cup Cheddar Cheese, Shredded

- 1 Teaspoon Onion Powder

- Sea Salt & Black Pepper to Taste

Directions:

1. Get out a skillet and place it over medium heat, and then melt your butter. Cook your onion for five minutes, stirring frequently.

2. Add in the cauliflower rice, and cook for another five minutes. Stir often to prevent burning.

3. Stir in your remaining ingredients, cooking until the cheese is melted. This should take three to five minutes, and serve warm.

STUFFED MUSHROOMS

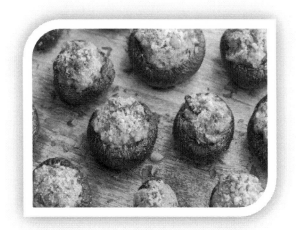

Serves: 4
Time: 30 Minutes
Calories: 270
Protein: 13 Grams
Fat: 20 Grams
Net Carbs: 7 Grams

Ingredients:

- 4 Portobello Mushrooms, Large & Stemmed

- 1 Tablespoon Olive Oil

- 10 Ounces Spinach, Frozen, Thawed, Drained & Chopped

- Sea Salt & Black Pepper to Taste

- 4 Ounces Cream Cheese, Room Temperature

- 14 Ounces Artichoke Hearts, Canned, Drained & chopped

- 1/4 Cup Sour Cream

- 1/2 Cup Mozzarella Cheese, Shredded

- 1 Teaspoon Garlic Powder

- 1/4 Cup Parmesan Cheese, Grated

Directions:

1. Start by heating your oven to 45, and then get out a baking sheet. Line it with foil, and then get your mushrooms. And then rub them with olive oil, seasoning with salt and pepper. Place them on the baking sheet, cooking for ten minutes. They should soften.

2. Ge tout a bowl and combine your mozzarella, spinach, cream cheese, sour cream, artichokes, garlic, salt and pepper.

3. Divide among your mushrooms, topping with parmesan. Bake for fifteen minutes. The filling should begin to bubble, and serve warm.

EASY CABBAGE

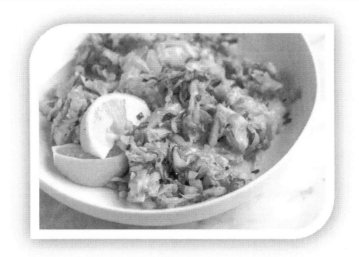

Serves: 4
Time: 20 Minutes
Calories: 158
Protein: 3 Grams
Fat: 12 Grams
Net Carbs: 7 Grams

Ingredients:

- 1/4 Cup Butter, Salted
- 3 Tablespoons Apple Cider Vinegar
- 1 Head Cabbage, Chopped
- Sea Salt & Black Pepper to Taste

Directions:

1. Start by getting out a stockpot, and then melt your butter over medium heat. Add in the cabbage, and cook. Stir occasionally, cooking until it's tender. It can take twelve to fifteen minutes.
2. Add in your remaining ingredients, and heat all the way through. Serve warm.

GREEK CUCUMBER SALAD

Serves: 6
Time: 15 Minutes
Calories: 590
Protein: 12 Grams
Fat: 55 Grams
Net Carbs: 10 Grams

Ingredients:

- 1/2 Cup Olive Oil
- 2 Tablespoons Red Wine Vinegar
- 1 Teaspoon Oregano
- 1 Teaspoon Garlic Salt
- Sea Salt & Black Pepper to Taste
- 4 Tomatoes, Diced
- 1 Red Onion, Sliced Thin
- 4 Cucumbers, Peeled, Sliced into Rounds & Quartered
- 1 Cup Feta Cheese, Crumbled
- 2 Cups Black Olives, Pitted &Sliced
- 2 Cups Pepperoni, Sliced & Halved

Directions:

1. Start by getting out a bowl and whisking your garlic, salt, pepper, oregano, oil and vinegar.
2. Get out another bowl and toss your cucumbers, tomatoes, olives, onion, cheese and salami together.
3. Pour in the dressing, and toss to coat before serving.

HOT SPINACH SALAD

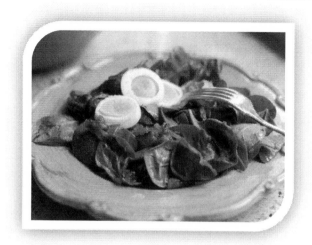

Serves: 6
Time: 25 Minutes
Calories: 265
Protein: 19 Grams
Fat: 18 Grams
Net Carbs: 4 Grams

Ingredients:

- 12 Slices Bacon, Uncured

- 1 Tablespoon Swerve

- 3 Tablespoons Apple Cider Vinegar

- 6 Cups Spinach, Fresh

- 1 Teaspoon Dijon Mustard

- 6 Hardboiled Eggs, Peeled & Sliced

- 1 Red Onion, Sliced Thin

- 2 Cups Mushrooms, Sliced

- 1 ½ Cups Swiss Cheese, Shredded

Directions:

1. Start by getting out a skillet and cooking your bacon over medium-low heat. Cook for about eight minutes or until it reaches the desired crispness. Line a plate with paper towels, and put your bacon slices on it to drain.

2. Use the bacon drippings to mix your sweetener, vinegar, and mustard, whisking until the swerve has dissolved. It should take about two minutes.

3. Divide your bacon, spinach, crumbles, egg, mushrooms, cheese, and onion among four bowls. Pour the mixture over top, and serve warm.

DESSERT RECIPES

LEMON COOKIES

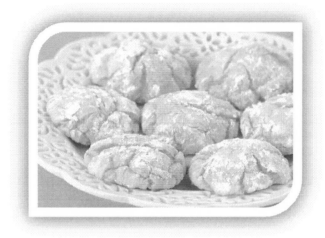

Serves: 12
Time: 20 Minutes
Calories: 140
Protein: 4 Grams
Fat: 9 Grams
Net Carbs: 4 Grams

Ingredients:

- 2 Eggs
- 1 Cup Cashew Butter
- 1/2 Teaspoon Vanilla Extract, Pure
- 10 Drops Liquid Stevia
- 1/4 Teaspoon Baking Soda
- 1 Lemon, Zested & Juiced

Directions:

1. Start by heating your oven to 350 and then get out two baking trays. Line them with parchment paper, and mix your eggs, baking soda, sweetener, vanilla and butter, lemon and sweetener together.

2. Roll the dough into balls, and then layer them on a baking tray. Sprinkle with lemon zest, and bake for twelve minutes.

COCONUT BITES

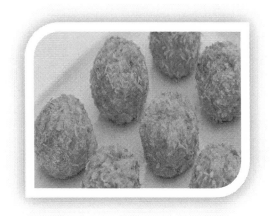

Serves: 4
Time: 10 Minutes
Calories: 644
Protein: 5 Grams
Fat: 65 Grams
Net Carbs: 7 Grams

Ingredients:

- 1 Cup Coconut Oil
- 1/2 Cup Chia Seeds
- 1 Teaspoon Vanilla Extract, Pure
- 1 Tablespoon Honey, Raw
- 1/4 Cup Coconut Flakes, Unsweetened

Directions:

1. Start by mixing all ingredients together, and then place them in the muffin tin. Place them in the freezer until you're ready to eat them.

5 MINUTE MOUSSE

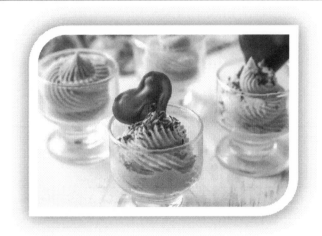

Serves: 4
Time: 5 Minutes
Calories: 222
Protein: 1 Gram
Fat: 22 Grams
Net Carbs: 4 Grams

Ingredients:

- 14 Ounces Coconut Cream, Canned & Chilled
- 1 Teaspoon Vanilla Extract, Pure
- 1/4 Cup Swerve
- 3 Tablespoons Cocoa Powder, Unsweetened

Directions:

1. Start by whipping your coconut cream with an electric mixture until fluffy.
2. Fold in your remaining ingredients, and serve immediately.

ALMOND FUDGE BROWNIES

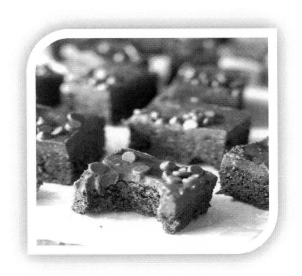

Serves: 16
Time: 15 Minutes
Calories: 118
Protein: 5 Grams
Fats: 11 Grams
Net Carbs: 5 Grams

Ingredients:

- 3/4 Cup Powdered Erythritol

- 3 Eggs, Large

- 1 Cup Almond Butter

- 10 Tablespoons Cocoa Powder, Unsweetened

- 1/2 Teaspoon Baking Powder

- Pinch Sea Salt

Directions:

1. Start by blending your erythritol and almond butter together. Add in the eggs, baking powder and cocoa before adding in your pinch of salt.

2. Once the batter is completely mixed, grease a nine by nine-inch baking pan and transfer your batter in it. smooth it out with a spatula, and bake at 325 for eleven minutes.

3. Allow it to cool for ten minutes before slicing.

PUMPKIN CHEESECAKE MOUSSE

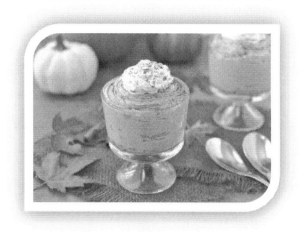

Serves: 10
Time: 15 Minutes
Calories: 215
Protein: 3 Grams
Fats: 18 Grams
Net Carbs: 3 Grams

Ingredients:

- 15 Ounces Pumpkin Puree, Canned & Unsweetened
- 12 Ounces Cream Cheese, Softened
- 2 Teaspoons Vanilla Extract, Pure
- 1/2 Cup Confectioners Erythritol
- 2 Tablespoons Pumpkin Pie Spice
- 3/4 Cup Heavy Cream

Directions:

1. Start by combining the pumpkin puree and cream cheese.
2. Once mixed add in your erythritol, vanilla extract, heavy cream and pumpkin pie spice. Mix until well combined.
3. Refrigerate for an hour before serving chilled.

DOUBLE CHOCOLATE MOUSSE

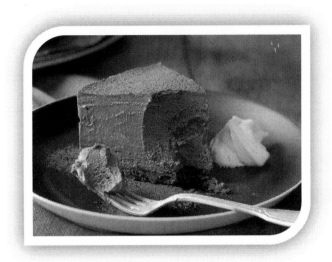

Serves: 2
Time: 25 Minutes
Calories: 461
Protein: 7 Grams
Fats: 45 Grams
Net Carbs: 5 Grams

Ingredients:

- 4 Ounces Cream Cheese

- 1 Cup Heavy Cream

- 1/4 Cup Powdered Erythritol

- 1 Ounce Chocolate Chips

- 2 Tablespoons Cocoa Powder

Directions:

1. Start by melting your chocolate chips over low heat in a pan, and then add in × cup of heavy cream.

2. Get out a bowl to beat your erythritol and cream cheese together.

3. Add in the cocoa powder and chocolate mixture, and then season with a pinch of salt. Beat until well combined, and then add in your remaining heavy cream. It should become whipped.

4. Prepare two bowls and layer before serving.

CONCLUSION

Now you have everything you need to get started on a successful ketogenic diet. With recipes that are under thirty minutes, it's easy to stick to the ketogenic diet and meet all your health and weight loss goals. Just remember the steps to success and start planning your meals so that you can stick to the diet easier. Avoid temptation at all costs when you're just getting started, and don't exercise your will power more than you must. While building up your will power will help you in the long run, if you subject yourself to too much temptation, you will eventually give in. pick a recipe, and get started on a journey to a happier, healthier you.

Made in the
USA
Columbia, SC